# Gagging For It

Cut yourself free from gagging with The Magic Technique™

Dr James Main

MAINBOYS
PUBLISHING

Mainboys Publishing

**Published by Mainboys Publishing**

**GAGGING FOR IT:**

**Cut yourself free from gagging with**

**The Magic Technique™**

***by* Dr James Main**





Printed Version ISBN: 978-1-0681959-0-7
eBook Version ISBN: 978-1-0681959-1-4

**Cover design and layout by:** Spiffing Publishing

To all my patients past and present that helped make the MAGIC happen

# Contents

# Introduction

The title of this book, *Gagging for It,* may make you think that it is either about experiencing something extremely desirable or about a group of people who are longing for something extremely desirable. In some ways, the latter is true, as this book is for the hundreds of millions of people around the world who suffer from hypersensitive premature gagging; they are literally gagging for a cure.

Published medical evidence suggests that if you experience hypersensitive premature gagging, then you are far from alone, as anything between 8% and 20%[1] of the population also suffers from this condition. Even if we take the lowest figure of 8%, this would mean that a staggering 650 million people suffer with this problem worldwide.

The condition can have a profound effect on their quality of life and also their ability to access medical and dental care. If you are one of the millions of people who has a hypersensitive premature gagging reflex, this book describes a simple procedure I have developed – called the MAGIC technique – that could cure you of this unfortunate affliction.

# Chapter One

# It's all about ME (Mind & Emotion)

I sometimes wonder what my parents must have thought of me as a child. I was born in Hong Kong in the early sixties and, from a young age, I loved to learn about science and the human psyche.

My two passions were atomic physics and hypnosis. So, instead of having posters on my wall of The Beatles, Paul Newman or Muhammed Ali, I made my own posters showing the movement of electrically charged particles through a magnetic field and I asked for the *Concise Encyclopaedia of the Atom* as my Christmas present.

Whilst this satisfied my passion for atomic physics, when it came to my passion for hypnosis, that was much harder to quench.

My desire to learn about hypnosis as a child was such that I remember one particular Christmas when my father and I went hunting all over Hong Kong for a book about it. We didn't find one, or at least not one suitable for a 10-year-old.

My interest in the human mind continued throughout school. I found that I quickly became the Agony Uncle for many of my fellow students, particularly the girls – which, for a teenage boy, was a double-edged sword!

Whilst I was at Edinburgh University studying dentistry, I became friendly with another student whose father was a psychiatrist and had taught him the mechanics of hypnosis, which my friend in turn taught me. I then practised hypnosis on my fellow students as an after-dinner party trick.

As soon as I qualified, I decided that I would like to learn about hypnosis and hypnotherapy for the treatment of my anxious patients and found that I was particularly adept at using this technique. At the time, I was a Dental Officer in the Royal Navy and quickly became skilled at practicing hypnosis on anxious sailors and marines. One extreme incident occurred when a sailor had his testicles knelt on by accident when mucking around with his mate and was in great pain. In the taxi taking him to our ship, in order to relieve his pain, I performed a "confusional" hypnotic technique on him which allowed him to walk up the gangway, whereas before he got in the taxi he could hardly stand up. This is one of the more difficult induction techniques.

During my time in the Royal Navy, whilst on seafaring duties I became aware that I was particularly good at understanding psychosomatic problems and then using hypnosis to cure them. One particular case has some relevance to gagging. A sailor was convinced that he had throat cancer, yet, despite all their medical investigations, the doctors said nothing could be found. During the consultation, I realised that the sailor had recently looked down his throat when he was very unwell with the flu, and had noticed the back of it was red with a white/greyish film over it, which he took for cancer, though in fact it was just phlegm.

Once I realised this was the problem, I was able to de-program this link through hypnosis, and he was not troubled with phantom throat cancer again.

When I left the Royal Navy in 1990, I became a dentist in Chester. I carried on with my hypnosis work in the evenings and became so good at it that, for a period of time in the 1990s, I was getting referrals from a consultant psychiatrist to treat psychosomatic disorders.

My treatment of patients with psychosomatic problems made me very aware of how the mind plays a very powerful role in how we respond to certain incidents that occur in our lives, especially at a young age, and how we can inadvertently develop problems which we are convinced have a physiological or pathological cause when they actually have a psychological origin from that earlier event.

One such incident that started me on this journey of finding a cause for psychogenic premature gagging was something that occurred to a friend of mine back in the 1990s. My friend, who was in his sixties, had seriously choked on a piece of bacon as an adult and afterwards had refused to eat bacon ever again. This seemed to me a little extreme for one incident that was unlikely to recur, but it did prompt me to think about why people gagged when I performed dental treatments yet could consume food and drinks without any problem whatsoever. It became clear to me that, for almost all my patients, this was not a physical problem but a psychosomatic condition; a powerful emotional link had been created to a moment when something in their mouths had caused a gagging response.

In addition to this realisation, over the past 15 years of treating patients with this issue, it has become clear to me that psychogenic hypersensitive gagging is not a gagging problem as such, but an airway problem. In other words, this emotional link is with an unpleasant experience in their early life, usually when they were a toddler, which involved difficulty breathing or the threat of suffocation, which is common in toddlers.

For some, this led to an overwhelming feeling of fear at the time of the incident as they were unable to rationalise it. In the toddler's mind, a link could have been made to their fear of something in their mouth or back of their throat and, once this link was established, it would lead to their hypersensitive gag reflex.

Once I established it was an airway problem, I started to investigate how psychologically expansive my patient's airway was, whether their hypersensitivity was just restricted to objects in the mouth or expanded beyond the mouth to other areas, such as round the neck and further. Initially, to my surprise, I found that virtually all the patients who suffered with hypersensitive gagging did not like wearing anything tight around their neck, and some would only wear loose clothing around their neck. I then wondered whether this hypersensitivity went even further and included their immediate personal 'airspace'. I asked them whether, if confronted with a crowded lift, they would wait for another one. In the majority of cases, the patient would say they would wait for another one, which lead to me to ask if they would go willingly into crowded or confined spaces and again most would say they would avoid such situations, which by definition is claustrophobia. This has led me to understand that, for a hypersensitive gagger, the anxiety and fear they experience when they feel their airway is threatened has greater ramifications than just gagging; unbeknownst to them, it can affect many aspects of their lives.

# Chapter Two

# Assessment of your gagging

In this chapter, I shall use a simple, points-based questionnaire for you to self-assess the severity of your hypersensitive gagging. Later in the book you will be able to use the points you scored to tailor the self-help cure for your gagging.

Before we go into the anatomy and physiology of gagging, you should take this simple multiple-choice questionnaire. Attached to each answer are points which, when added up, will indicate the severity of your gag reflex.

***

**Are you able to brush your back teeth or the back of your palate without gagging?**

*Yes* – 0 point
*No* – 2 points

**Are you able to undergo dental procedures without gagging?**

*Yes* – 1 point

*No* – 2 points
*Have not been to the dentist* – 0 points

**To avoid gagging, are you only able to insert a fork or chopsticks into the front of your mouth?**

*Yes* – 2 points
*No* – 0 points

**Do you avoid wearing tight clothing around your neck, such as neckties and scarves?**

*Yes* – 2 points
*No* – 0 point

**Do you avoid going into crowded spaces?**

*Yes* – 2 points
*No* – 0 point

**Would you say you suffer with claustrophobia?**

*Yes* – 2 points
*No* – 0 point

*0 - 1 point:* You do not have a hypersensitive premature gag reflex

*2 - 5 points:* You have a mild to moderate hypersensitive premature gag reflex

*6 – 9 points:* You have a moderate to severe hypersensitive premature gag reflex

*10 – 12 points:* You have a severe hypersensitive premature gag reflex

If you have scored two or more points in the questionnaire above, then this book is for you. The higher your score, the more the MAGIC technique will help to transform your quality of life.

## Now for some medical stuff

It is difficult to draw a distinct line between normal - or "somatic" - gagging, triggered by stimulation at the back of the throat, and "psychogenic gagging", which is a gag reflex triggered by psychological or emotional factors. This explains why some people are able to brush their teeth and eat and drink with no issues but have trouble wearing dentures or having dental X-rays taken without gagging. Other factors such as gastrointestinal issues and other medical conditions, hypersensitivity associated with heavy smoking, alcoholism, anatomic abnormalities, and anxiety disorders can all contribute to an exaggerated or hypersensitive gag reflex.

Generally, somatic gagging is triggered by physical contact at the back of the mouth, tongue, tonsils, and throat which induces contractions to initiate gagging and retching. This is a natural response to prevent choking or food entering the windpipe or lungs. By contrast, psychogenic gagging can be triggered not only by physical contact but also by smells, sights, anxiety, and even thoughts – such as thinking about having dental impressions taken.

The gag reflex is mediated by the glossopharyngeal sensory nerve and the vagus motor nerve. The roots of these nerves connect the muscle at the back of the throat, the soft palate, the rear third of the tongue, upper part of the throat, and a part of the brain known as the medulla.

There are many physical and psychological factors that can affect a person's gag reflex. The reflex, especially a hyperactive one, can be triggered or exacerbated by psychological conditions. Anxiety, for example, often leads to people having a heightened awareness to physical sensations in their body as well as increased muscle tension. These symptoms combined can make people more reactive to any sensations in the mouth or throat and, in turn, to the threat of psychogenic gagging. Anxiety can trigger the gagging response this way, in turn increasing the level of anxiety, creating a vicious gagging cycle.

Physical factors affecting the gag reflex range from gastrointestinal (gut) conditions such as acid reflux and gastritis (inflammation of the stomach lining) to anatomical features like a deviated (off-centre) nasal septum, and neurological disorders.

There is no one cause for gagging but in this book, we are addressing psychogenic gagging – also known as hypersensitive premature gagging – where there is no physical or pathological cause.

In the following chapters, I will describe existing treatments, explain how my experience as a dentist has led me to reach a surprising conclusion about the cause of gagging – and propose a simple but effective new treatment that could eliminate the problem completely.

## Chapter Three

# Current cures for hypersensitive gagging

There are numerous treatments and interventions that can alleviate psychogenic gagging, including:

1. Sedative and anaesthetic drugs.
2. Acupuncture and/or acupressure.
3. Distraction techniques, including the use of VR (virtual reality) glasses.
4. Cognitive behavioural therapy.

Many studies have assessed the effectiveness of sedatives and anaesthetics to reduce the gag reflex. These include a trial of the efficacy of a sedative called propofol when used alone versus propofol administered in combination with another sedative called midazolam[2]. The authors of this study reported a reduction in the gag reflex. However, propofol is known to cause loss of memory of events, and patients under the influence of midazolam are unable to create new short-term memories. While such drugs may be effective to help with one episode of medical or dental treatment, they do not address the causes of the gag reflex, and so they need to be administered again whenever it might be a problem. This is not ideal as sedatives and anaesthetics are not only costly, but they come with their own risks.

How about alternative medicine? Studies have shown that techniques such as acupuncture, acupressure, and hypnosis have varying levels of success, and their authors suggest that a more holistic approach is often necessary due to the multitude of factors that can affect a gag reflex. Acupuncture has long been investigated as a way to reduce the reflex and studies have produced largely positive results. While this may be a useful technique for some, it requires an acupuncturist and does not provide a permanent cure. On top of this, if you already have an aversion to needles, it is unlikely acupuncture is going to relax you during preparation for dental treatment.

Distraction techniques, including the use of virtual reality (VR) headsets, have shown mixed results. Some people are more responsive to these methods than others. However, as they do not address the cause of gagging, they provide transient relief at best.

Similarly, cognitive behavioural therapy (CBT) can be useful in reducing anxiety by changing your thought patterns, and therefore your emotional reactions, to lessen the psychogenic gag reflex. This is not a foolproof method, however, as CBT can take a long time before you see any changes and, as with the distraction techniques, some people are more receptive than others.

Attempting just to treat the symptoms of a psychogenic gag reflex often proves fruitless. Instead, I recommend addressing the cause with a simple self-help method that over time can provide a permanent cure. This is what the MAGIC technique provides.

# Chapter Four

# Why do you have a hypersensitive gag reflex?

Choking is a leading cause of a reduction in the quality of health and even mortality amongst toddlers[3]. When a toddler experiences a choking episode, they do not have the cognitive ability to understand what is actually happening, but they do experience overwhelming fear. All toddlers operate on an emotional level and not on a cognitive, analytical level. I believe that for many of them, an important link is then made between having something in their mouth, which caused the choking, and a deep-seated experience of fear which could be as severe as a near death experience. Once that link has established itself, then every time that person has something in their mouth which is not food or drink, it triggers that fearful emotion, causing them to gag in order to expel that foreign object from their mouth.

It was my experience of using hypnosis when dealing with entrenched psychosomatic disorders, as well as my friend giving me an insight into his rejection of eating bacon (see page 8), that prompted me to realise that psychogenic hypersensitive gagging was an airway problem and not a gagging problem. If hypersensitive gagging were a reflex to protect the gullet, then the people that suffer with it would be extremely thin as they would not be able to swallow food. I could see from my patients that none of them were suffering with starvation, which again led me to believe that this is an airway problem. Because of this understanding, from now on in this book I shall no longer use the term 'psychogenic hypersensitive gagging' but instead will use the term 'psychogenic airway protection' or PAP.

In order to fully understand and treat PAP, you need to accept that this is an airway problem and not simply a gagging problem. You also need to realise that all the air from the opening of your mouth right through to the minor bronchioles (the smallest air tubes) in your lungs is completely useless until it reaches the alveoli, which are the structures where oxygen and carbon dioxide are exchanged between the blood in your circulatory system and the outside world. The air that you have in your mouth and the network of tubes in your lungs is only there to transport these gases to and from the alveoli. It is known as the tidal volume. It is also important to understand that, once the link has been established between something in your mouth that is not food or drink and the emotions that you experience – whether it's initially anxiety or full-on fear – it will be reinforced each time you gag and reject that foreign object. This further strengthens the link that was created when you were a toddler.

What the MAGIC technique does is to give you a tool to decouple that link and break the cycle of fear and gagging. This can be for short-term relief of the symptoms, in order to conduct a specific medical procedure or to prevent you from reacting to something in your mouth for a short while, or it can be combined with desensitisation to break that link over time so that you can, from then on, tolerate having objects in your mouth without triggering the learned emotional response.

This will lead to a profound improvement in your quality of life by allowing you to undergo medical and dental procedures that were intolerable before, wear neckties, buttoned up collars or scarves, and even go into crowded spaces without feeling claustrophobic and take up activities that you would not have considered such as snorkelling or other water sports.

In the next chapter I explain how hypersensitive gagging can impact your life beyond the dentist's chair, and provide a step-by-step guide to overcoming it.

## Chapter Five

# The MAGIC technique

Once you recognise that the cause of your gagging, or PAP, is an airway problem as opposed to a gagging problem – which to you seems like a normal response to having an object in your mouth other than something you can eat or drink – then the question becomes how do you switch this link off, based on there being a psychological link between the need to protect your airway and your urge to gag.

I have found that the longer someone has lived with this problem, the worse it gets. This is logical, as every time the sufferer has something placed in their mouth other than food and drink, or attempts to wear clothing around their neck, it causes them to gag immediately or feel very uncomfortable, and this then reinforces the psychogenic link that was established in their childhood. Any desensitization to eliminate the link is not going to happen with just one session at the dentist using the MAGIC technique but will require a determined effort to gradually erode and ultimately eliminate this link.

Gagging may also have wider effects beyond the dentist. For example, if you can't wear a tie this could have an impact on the jobs you can do or how you present yourself at important occasions in your life such as weddings or funerals. It may also have an impact on the types of spaces that you feel comfortable in. Many people who have hypersensitive gagging find being in small, crowded places, or even going into areas that they perceive to be crowded, makes them feel claustrophobic. This may mean that they are unable to go into elevators or crowded venues such as pubs. This could have all sorts of social and work ramifications, as well as restricting their ability to go about their day without the fear or anxiety about finding themself in such a space.

I developed MAGIC (which stands for Main Amelioration for Gagging Indoctrination by

Communication) to help people who experience these everyday problems. The technique involves using a physiological phenomenon whereby taking a deep breath causes stretch receptors in your lungs to send an extremely strong signal to the respiratory centre of the brain. This signal tells the brain that you have plenty of air in your lungs and there is nothing to worry about. This effect has been proven in both physiological experiments on animals as well as in human beings[4,5]. As a result of the signal from the lungs that everything is ok, the central nervous system effectively switches off the gag reflex.

## Short term solution

If you have a hypersensitive gag response and you need to have a dental X-ray or some other procedure that involves something being placed in your mouth, there is a simple, short-term solution. First, ask the clinician not to put anything in your mouth until you are ready, which you will signal by opening your mouth. Before that happens, take a big breath that will stretch your lungs, then open your mouth to allow the clinician to place whatever object is required in your mouth. During the procedure it is important that you do not hold your breath but breathe deeply. With each inhalation you will stretch your lungs, triggering the stretch receptors each time, thereby providing a regular signal to your respiratory centres to allow you to feel comfortable throughout the procedure.

By practising this simple technique, you will be able to overcome the short-term effects of your hypersensitive gagging reflex in order to undergo any procedure where having an object in your mouth is required.

I have treated hundreds of patients this way. I usually only discover that someone has this hypersensitive reflex when I try to place an X-ray sensor in their mouth and they gag and spit it out. I then explain to them that it is an airway problem and not a gagging problem as such (related to swallowing) and describe how the little trick of stretching their lungs before I place the X-ray sensor in their mouth will negate their gag reflex. I ask them to open their mouths only after they have done this. Needless to say, everyone is sceptical at first but then, without fail, after the X-ray has been taken successfully, they are all amazed at the MAGIC of doing something they had never been able to do before.

## Long term solution and cure

The hypersensitive gag reflex can have profound effects on your quality of life, to the extent that you may avoid certain situations. You may be unwilling or even feel unable to undergo particular medical or dental procedures, to wear the clothing that you need to in certain situations, such as job interviews or formal social occasions, and even struggle to take a shower. This can have an impact on your self-esteem, your general health and wellbeing, and your overall confidence in navigating the world.

An example of this is what happened to a patient I treated called Roger.

Roger came to me with such severe disease in all his remaining teeth and gums that all of his remaining teeth had to be removed. The problem was that Roger had a severe hypersensitive gag reflex, so he was unable to tolerate having an upper denture to replace all his top teeth and cover his whole palate. I advised him that the solution would be upper and lower implant retained bridges, which would avoid introducing a foreign object at the back of his palate. Unfortunately, Roger did not have the financial resources to have this treatment option, the only alternative being full upper and lower dentures after all the diseased teeth had been extracted and his gums had fully healed.

I used the MAGIC technique to help me to take the moulds for the upper and lower dentures, but, more importantly, I explained to Roger how he could chip away at it and eventually eliminate the learned response that was the cause of his PAP.

By the time I came to fit the dentures, which was about 8 weeks from when I advised Roger on how to use the MAGIC technique, he was able to tolerate a full upper and lower denture, despite the back of the full upper denture extending to the back of his palate.

When I rang Roger 6 months after fitting the dentures to see how he was getting on, he said they were working really well and, when I asked him about his gagging, it turned out he had almost forgotten that he was a gagger at all!

If you are willing to make an effort in order to cure yourself of the hypersensitive gag response, which was probably established when you were a toddler, then it has to be done with a combination of the MAGIC technique and desensitisation. Before deciding which is the best starting point for this process, you need to refer to the score that you achieved earlier in this book in the questionnaire to determine the severity of your hypersensitive psychogenic gagging (see page 10).

## Scoring 2 to 5 points: Mild to moderate hypersensitive premature gag reflex

If you fall into this category, most of your hypersensitive gag response is based around foreign objects in your mouth only. The long-term cure for all hypersensitive premature gagging is to erode and desensitise the conditioned link between having something in your mouth and the psychogenic airway protection response (see page 19).

Using the MAGIC technique, you will need to do the following:

Have a toothbrush ready and stand in front of a mirror.

## Method A

1. Fill your lungs with air so that they are fully stretched, place the toothbrush towards the back of your mouth to a point where you would normally not be able to go without gagging, then remove the toothbrush from your mouth. Do this at least 10 times to show that this is not a one off and that you can repeat the process without gagging. If at any stage of this procedure you do feel that you are about to gag, remove the toothbrush from your mouth, then again take a deep breath to stretch your lungs and put the toothbrush straight back to where it was before. You will find that this cancels the effects of your desire to gag.

2. Practice taking a big breath in, with each inhalation stretching your lungs, and then breathing out, followed by another big breath in to stretch your lungs before breathing out again. These should be large, steady inhalations with each one stretching your lungs to their full extent.

3. In front of a mirror, take the same breaths as above and, at the same time, place the toothbrush to a point at the back of your mouth where you would normally find it would make you gag. It is important that whilst you are doing this you are following the breathing patterns as previously explained in point 2.

4. Keep the toothbrush at the back of your mouth for at least 2 breaths then take it out.

5. Repeat point 4 until you feel comfortable with the toothbrush in your mouth and then increase the number of breaths that you are able to take prior to taking the toothbrush out. The aim is to be able to take at least 10 breaths and still feel comfortable with the toothbrush in place at the back of your mouth.

6. Once you are able to take 10 breaths, as described above, move the toothbrush across the palate from one side to the other side whilst taking deep, slow breaths but always being aware of the fullness of air in your lungs, stretching the lungs

further if necessary

7. Keep practising the deep breathing procedure while moving the toothbrush around until you can breathe normally, with maybe an occasional deep breath if you feel a sudden urge to gag.

The more that this final process is practised, the more you will unlearn the link that is causing the premature hypersensitive gagging, until you have eroded it to such an extent that there is no longer a psychogenic link.

## Scoring 6 to 12 points: Moderate to severe hypersensitive premature gag reflex

For people with a moderate to severe, or a severe premature gag reflex, it would be too much to start treatment within the mouth. Rather, treatment should start more gradually, around the neck. However, the process of eroding the link follows the same principles as for people with a mild to moderate premature gag reflex.

For this process you can use either a scarf or a necktie and do the following:

## Method B

1. Place the scarf or necktie loosely around your neck and stand in front of a mirror.

2. Before starting to tighten the necktie or scarf, take a big breath to stretch your lungs and then tighten the necktie or scarf for no more than one or two seconds. In normal circumstances you might find that this is quite uncomfortable and may even initiate a gag response. However, by doing it in this manner you should find that whilst your lungs are inflated there is no gag response and you should generally feel comfortable.

3. Once you have done this several times, so that you feel quite comfortable when tightening your necktie or scarf around your neck for 2 seconds, you should extend the time with the scarf or necktie firmly around your neck and take steady and deep breaths. With each breath you take in, you will stretch your lungs. Do not hold your breath, as this is counter-productive, but your

breathing should be steady and deep. If at any point you feel uncomfortable, loosen the necktie or scarf and start again.

4. When you are able to keep the necktie or scarf around your neck for at least a minute without feeling uncomfortable, you can gradually decrease the intensity of your breathing until you are breathing normally. However, if at any stage you feel uncomfortable then return to the more intensive breathing where you are inflating your lungs to their greatest extent to counteract the discomfort that you are experiencing. You can then gradually return to normal breathing again.

5. The ultimate test for the full erosion or elimination of the link that has caused your gagging would be to wear a necktie or scarf for several hours without feeling any particular discomfort.

6. Once you have achieved point five, you should then proceed to the next stage, which is eliminating the gagging problem when you have

objects in your mouth. This should be done by following the procedure as laid out above under the heading 'Scoring 2 to 5 points: Mild to moderate hypersensitive premature gag reflex'.

For those of you who scored 10 to 12 points in the earlier questionnaire, once you have completed Methods A and B successfully, you will then need to experience what it feels like either to go into a crowded space or into an elevator. If at any time you start feeling uncomfortable, then go back to the breathing procedure as laid out in Method A, Point 2.

To test that you have truly eliminated the psychogenic link that you have carried for so many years, you should be able to go into these spaces and find the experience at least tolerable, if not entirely comfortable.

In the next chapter of the book, I will explore the impact hypersensitive gagging has had on the patients I have treated, not only in the dental setting but also how it has affected their lives and how the MAGIC technique has helped improve their quality of life in ways that I had not considered.

# Chapter Six

# The Gaggers

Over the years I have treated many patients for their PAP with almost 100% success. The most common scenario is that I initially explain the reasons why they have this problem – and that it is an airway problem and not a gagging problem per se – and ask them to take a big breath and stretch their lungs before I place an X-ray sensor into their mouth. I say they should only open their mouths to receive the X-ray sensor once they have filled their lungs up. Many are skeptical that they will not gag but are happy to follow my advice as I am their dentist. However, after I have taken the X-ray, some are pleasantly surprised that they did not gag, and some are absolutely amazed as they have never had X-rays taken without gagging and assume that the reflex is just part of their make-up.

I had a stark example of how people who gag think that this is not only normal for them, but normal for everyone else. I was meeting my financial adviser and her colleague – let us call them Jane and Ann. In the course of the meeting, I spoke to them about this book to discuss the financial implications of the possible income. I described what the book was about and asked if either of them tends to gag at the dentist, to which Ann replied that she did. When Jane said that she did not, Ann was amazed. "I thought everyone gagged at the dentist," she said. These two women had worked together for many years and clearly this was something that they did not know about each other.

This conversation generated two thoughts for me. First, gaggers do not think it is abnormal to gag, especially when at the dentist, and second, that it is not something that is discussed.

If a hypersensitive gag reflex were just a problem when you were at the dentist's and having an examination of the back of your throat, then it would not be worth my while to write a book about it. The academic paper I published in *The British Dental Journal* would suffice. However, many years ago I wondered whether, if this was an airway problem, it extended beyond the actual airway to clothing or items around the neck and even to being in crowded places? To test this hypothesis, I asked patients who were gaggers if they liked to wear tight clothing around their neck, such as a necktie or a polo neck jumper. Almost every patient I asked would tell me that they chose not to wear tight clothing around their neck and many of them avoided crowded situations or were even claustrophobic. This became such a common answer that I stopped asking the question but instead I now say to patients who gag: "You probably do not like to wear tight clothing around your neck or go into crowded rooms or lifts." They are often quite surprised at my insight into their behaviour!

I remember one patient in particular who was a severe gagger. After I had gone through the MAGIC technique with him and taken the X-rays, he told me that he wished he had seen me years before. He explained that he had fallen out with his brother because when his brother got married all the other groomsmen were in suits and ties, but he had refused to wear a tie. This caused quite an upset at the time and had marred their relationship.

I have had patients who are in their 70s and have suffered with gagging all their adult lives. One woman – let us call her Sarah – told me that earlier in her life she had lived in Singapore, which has a lot of high-rise buildings, and she found it very uncomfortable to go into lifts. I went through the MAGIC technique with Sarah, which she went on to practice by herself at home. One of the unforeseen benefits was that Sarah was able to wash her hair under the shower for the first time. This showed me that the possible quality-of-life benefits gained by using the MAGIC technique have yet to be fully explored.

In Chapter 5, I wrote about Roger to demonstrate that the MAGIC technique will cure your gagging, but more importantly, that you will experience many other benefits, some of which I currently do not know myself.

I wait for you, the reader, to tell me!

## Chapter Seven

# The Evidence

If you have got to this part of the book, you have probably either experienced the instant relief the MAGIC technique has given you, or you have persevered to achieve the long-term cure.

However, if you have done neither and still remain skeptical, then you should read my paper *"Main amelioration of gagging indoctrination by communication - a MAGIC technique"* published in *The British Dental Journal* on 26 April 2024.

You can also view the YouTube video of me treating a patient with a severe gag reflex while taking a mould of their teeth.

*BDJ* MAGIC paper

https://www.nature.com/articles/s41415-024-7285-z

Patient gagging when I place an impression tray in their mouth.

https://youtube.com/shorts/8FeJmb4nUG0

Patient not gagging because of the MAGIC technique.

https://youtu.be/cvAm-cr1__E

I hope that you persevere and manage to cure your gag reflex through the MAGIC technique and achieve the quality of life you wish for.

# About the Author

Dr James Main has been a practicing private dentist for the past 40 years, working in the UK and overseas. He was a Royal Navy Dental Officer and taught for many years at the University of Manchester Dental School. He currently works at his private dental practice in Somerset, where he lives with his family and their dog.

He is the co-author of several academic papers in dental journals, both in the UK and the US, and is also a published poet.

Dr James has had a lifelong interest in hypnotherapy, successfully treating numerous patients for psychosomatic disorders unrelated to dentistry.

He has spent the last 15 years developing the MAGIC technique and in 2024 published a paper about it in *The British Dental Journal* for the benefit of other clinicians.

# References

1. Zafersoy akarslan, Zühre. GAG REFLEX IN DENTISTRY: WHAT CAN WE DO?. *Atatürk Üniversitesi Diş Hekimliği Fakültesi Dergisi.* 2016; 503-503. 10.17567/ataunidfd.290426.

2. Yamamoto T, Fujii-Abe K, Fukayama H, Kawahara H. The Effect of Adding Midazolam to Propofol Intravenous Sedation to Suppress Gag Reflex During Dental Treatment. *Anesthesia Progress.* 2018;**65**(2):76–81.

3. Levin RA, Smith GA. Choking Prevention Among Young Children. *Pediatric Annals.* 2010;**39**(11):721–4.

4. Chaffee RB, Zabara J, Tansy MF. Suppression of the Gag Reflex by Exaggerated Respiratory Movements. *Journal of Dental Research.* 1970;**49**(3):572–5.

5. Fowler WS. Breaking Point of Breath-Holding. *Journal of Applied Physiology.* 1954;**6**(9):539–45.

www.ingramcontent.com/pod-product-compliance
Lightning Source LLC
LaVergne TN
LVHW022030200926
848481LV00007B/2619
* 9 7 8 1 0 6 8 1 9 5 9 0 7 *